ICU Diary

for families

A Guided Resource for
Reflections, Medical Notes,
and Healing Together

Nicole Cromwell, MSN, RN

Copyright © 2025 Nicole Cromwell, MSN, RN
All Rights Reserved

Published by Nicole Cromwell, MSN, RN
Carmel, California

Print ISBN: 979-8-9992543-0-6

All rights reserved. No part of this publication may be reproduced, stored in a retrieval system, or transmitted in any form or by any means, electronic, mechanical, photocopying, recording, or otherwise, without prior written permission from the author, except for brief quotations used in reviews or academic work.

This journal was created as a supportive companion during hospitalization. A space for reflection, emotional processing, and personal notes. It is not intended to replace medical advice, diagnosis, or treatment, nor to serve as official medical documentation. Please consult your healthcare team for clinical decisions. If you are feeling overwhelmed or emotionally distressed, please speak with your care team or a mental health professional. Support is available.

Cover photo and interior artwork by Nicole Cromwell.

ICUDiary.com
Hospitalwellnessjournal.com
Nicolecromwellart.com

Printed in the United States of America on acid-free paper

This journal is a place for reflection, connection, and hope, a companion to guide you through this journey.

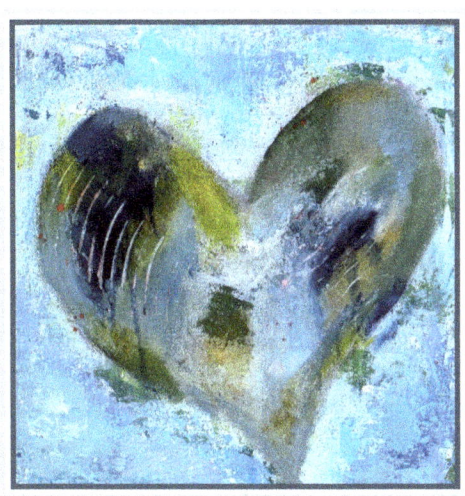

This journal belongs to:

_____

If found please call:

_____

Your Care Partner & Emergency Contact

It's important to have someone you trust to support you during your hospital stay. This person, often called a Care Partner or Emergency Contact, can help you communicate with the medical team, keep track of important updates, and support your care decisions. Many hospitals will ask for this information upon admission.

To avoid confusion, consider designating one primary contact person to receive updates and share them with others as needed. This helps ensure clear and consistent communication.

If you've named someone to make healthcare decisions for you, called a Durable Power of Attorney for Healthcare (DPOA), be sure to let your care team know. This person can speak on your behalf if you're ever unable to make decisions for yourself due to illness or injury. If you don't have a DPOA in place, most hospitals can help you complete the paperwork during your stay.

You can ask a nurse, social worker, or case manager for help.

Tip: It's helpful to share this contact information with close family or friends so everyone stays informed and communication remains clear.

Primary Care Partner / Emergency Contact:
Name: _____
Relationship: _____
Phone Number: _____

☐ This person is my Durable Power of Attorney for Healthcare (DPOA)

Optional Secondary Contact:
Name: _____
Relationship: _____
Phone Number: _____

Visiting Hours: _____

Room Number: _____

Important Phone Numbers

Main Hospital: _____

Nursing Station: _____

Reception: _____

Social Worker: _____

Chaplain/Spiritual Care: _____

Patient Information Desk: _____

Other: _____

_____

_____

_____

_____

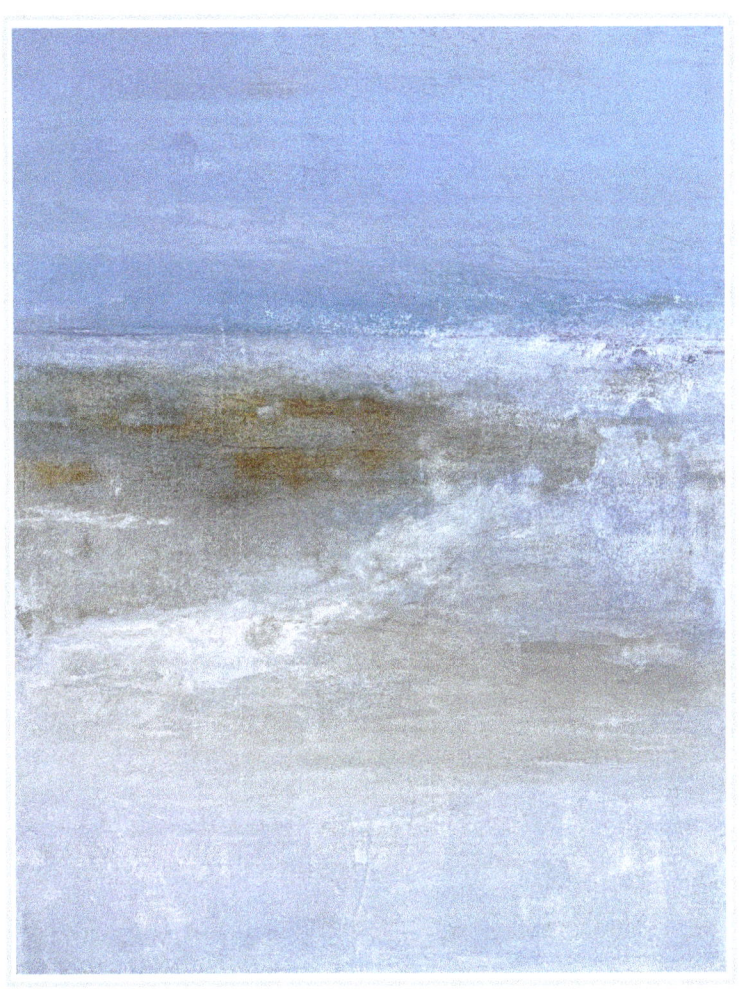

I plod, I ponder. Some days I simply exist.

- Paul Kalanithi, MD
When Breath Becomes Air

Table of Contents

Welcome to the ICU Diary for Families 1

Daily Updates & Questions for the Medical Team 4

Caring for Yourself During a Hospital Stay 31

Messages and Notes for Your Loved Ones 50

Patient Reflections 64

Hospital Support Services Available During Your Stay 72

After the ICU: Continuing Recovery With This Diary 75

A Note of Gratitude 77

"Getting to Know Me" 79

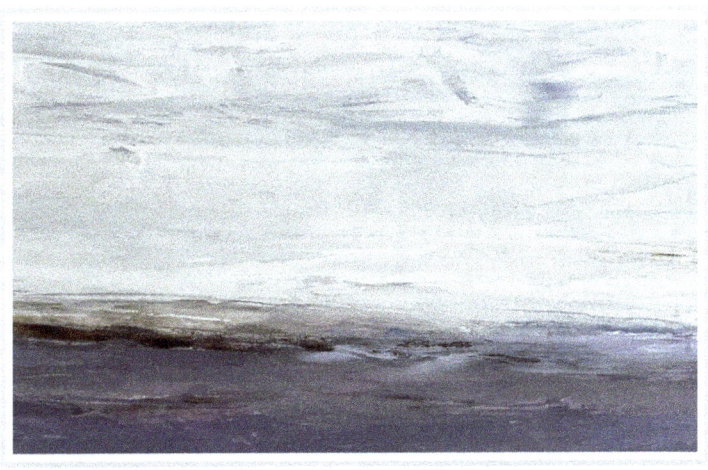

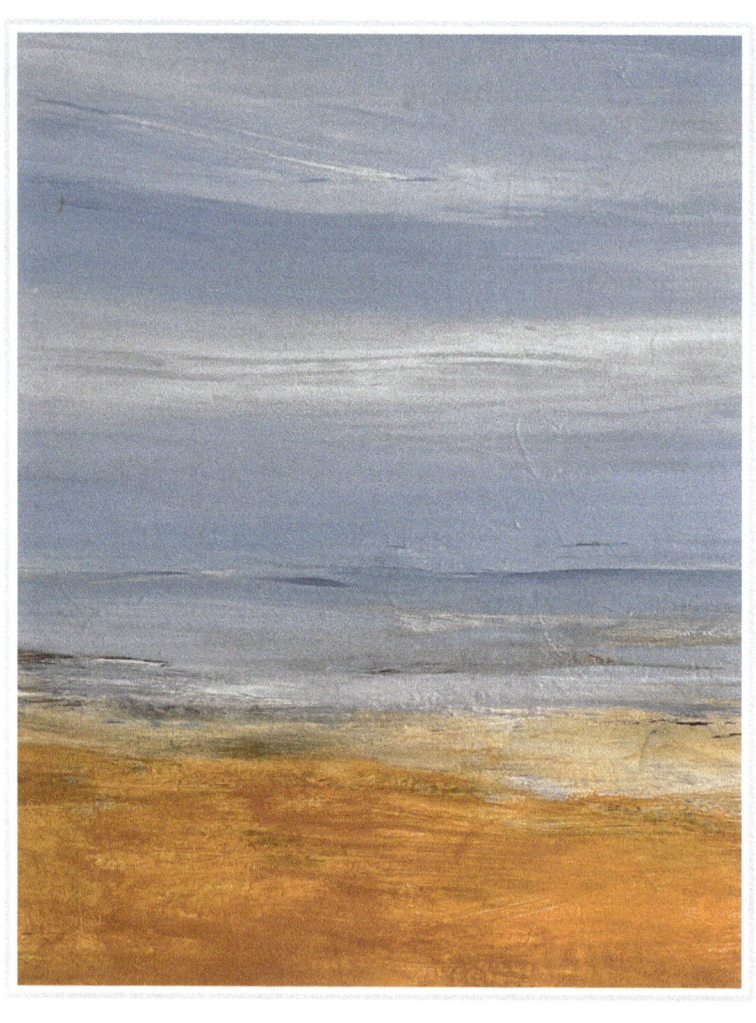

*Even the smallest acts of love and care
can spark hope.*

- Unknown

Welcome to the ICU Diary for Families

This journal has been thoughtfully created to support you and your loved one during this challenging time. Having a family member in the ICU can bring moments of uncertainty, complex medical information, and a wide range of emotions, which can feel overwhelming.

Patients often have little or no memory of their ICU stay due to medications or illness, which can lead to confusion, distress, or vivid dreams and hallucinations that feel very real. These experiences, along with physical and emotional challenges after discharge, can contribute to Post-Intensive Care Syndrome (PICS). While PICS doesn't affect everyone, it may include memory issues, anxiety, depression, or physical weakness in patients. Families can also experience PICS, with emotional distress or difficulty processing their loved one's ICU journey.

This journal is a supportive tool for tracking daily events, reflecting on experiences, and offering clarity and reassurance. It can help patients understand their time in the ICU and provide families with a way to process their own emotions. Reviewing the diary together can be a meaningful step in the healing process fostering understanding, connection, and recovery for both patients and their loved ones. By documenting these moments, the diary becomes not only a tool for healing but also a keepsake of resilience, strength, and hope through this difficult time.

Your voice, experiences, and well-being matter.
This journal is here to help you stay informed, connected,
and supported every step of the way.

A Note for Families & Staff

This journal is not a legal or medical document. It's a personal tool designed to offer comfort, track progress, and foster connection.

Taking an active role in care can help you feel more engaged and confident. Here are some helpful questions you might ask the nursing staff:

- What is the daily routine, and what should we expect?
- Are there specific visiting guidelines or ways we can participate in care?
- What can we do to support comfort and recovery?
- When do daily rounds usually take place?
- What time is shift change?

How Family and Friends Can Help in the ICU

Small, familiar actions can bring comfort and connection.

- Speak in a calm, clear voice.
- Remind them of the day and date.
- Talk about family, friends, or familiar memories.

For anything you bring into the room or play for your loved one, please check with the care team first.

- Glasses, hearing aids, or dentures
- Photos, calendars, or small familiar items
- Favorite music or TV shows

If your loved one is experiencing delirium, the care team may ask you to sit with them and offer reassurance.

Getting Started: How to Use This Journal

- **Daily Updates:** Track updates on your loved one's condition, treatments, progress, and reflections.
- **Questions for the Medical Team:** Write down questions for doctors or nurses and record answers to stay informed and organized
- **Emotional Reflections and Coping Strategies:** Use this space to process thoughts, practice gratitude, and record positive moments of hope or strength.
- **Messages and Notes for Your Loved One**: Write messages of encouragement and support for your family member. Share these notes during or after recovery, offering comfort and insight into this journey.
- **Patient Reflections:** If your loved one is awake and able to communicate, they can share thoughts and experiences, creating a personal record of their journey.
- **Support Resources:** Provides an overview of resources for families during an ICU stay, including spiritual care, social work, and case management.
- **Optional Gratitude Notes:** Use this page to write a thank-you note for someone who made a difference in your care. Tear it out and give it to a staff member as a simple way to share your appreciation.
- **Getting to Know Me Template:** An optional template to share your personal details about your loved one with the ICU team, such as their preferred name, hobbies, and favorite music. This helps staff connect beyond the patient's medical needs.

Daily Updates & Questions for the Medical Team

This section is designed to support reflection, connection, and healing, both during and after the ICU stay. Revisiting what you've written can help you acknowledge the progress made and better understand the journey as it unfolds. While recovery has its challenges, this journal offers space for expression and serves as a meaningful record of resilience and growth.

There's no right or wrong way to use it.

Write as much or as little as feels helpful, whether it's noting medical updates, capturing small moments of hope, or simply tracking the day's events. You don't need to write every day. Even brief entries can bring clarity, comfort, and perspective.

If multiple people are taking turns at the beside, this journal can also serve as a communication bridge, helping everyone stay informed, involved, and connected, even when they can't be there in person.

The next section includes twelve days of paired pages: one side for condition updates, the other for questions you may want to ask the care team. If your loved one's stay extends beyond this, consider continuing with a blank notebook or journal of your choice. The practice of writing, no matter where it continues, can offer support and insight throughout the healing process.

General Questions for the Medical Team

These questions are suggestions only and may not apply every day. If you're unsure what to ask, your nurse can help guide you. **Nurses are a wealth of knowledge** and can help you focus on what is most important for the patient's care.

About the Condition

- What is the current diagnosis or concern?
- How is progress being tracked?
- What specific goals should we focus on?

About Treatments and Procedures

- What treatments or procedures are planned?
- What side effects might occur, and how are they managed?
- When can we expect to see results?
- Are other options available?

About Daily Care

- What is the plan of care for today or tomorrow?
- How can we enhance comfort or manage discomfort?
- What milestones should we aim for (e.g., mobility, eating)?
- Are there activities or therapies to support recovery?

About Long-Term Plans

- What's the nest step when progress is made?
- Are there signs to watch for during recovery?
- Will there be special care needs after discharge?
- What resources are available to help with the transition?
- If we don't see the progress we hope for, what other options or support are available?

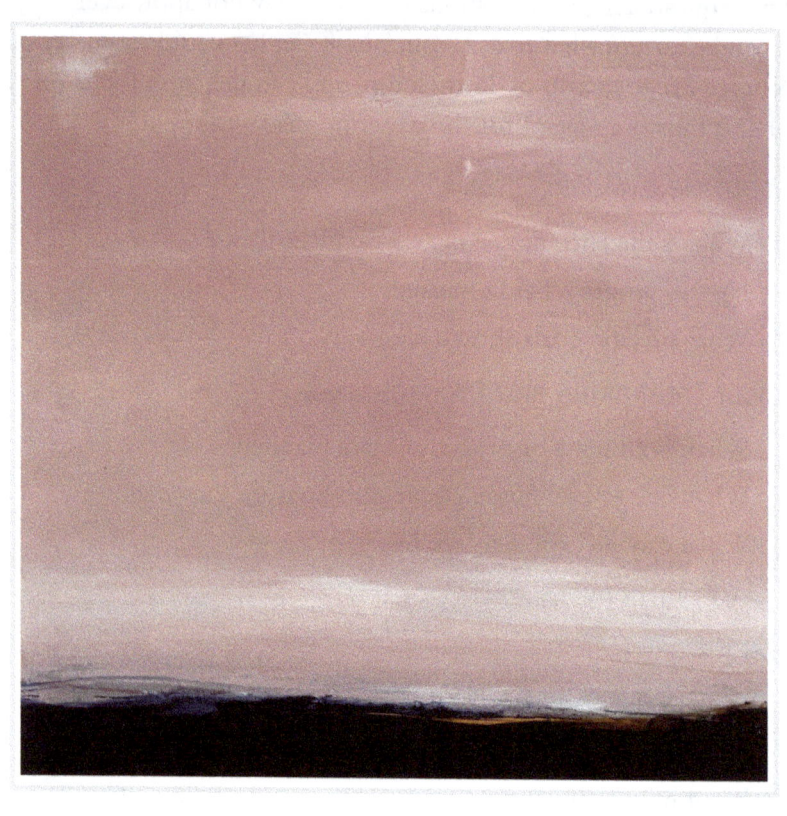

*Hope is the light that guides us through
the darkest days.*

- Unknown

Questions to Support Communication and Emotional Well-Being

It's okay to have questions, not just about treatments or test results, but also about how you're feeling and how to stay connected to the care team.

This page offers thoughtful questions you can ask to help you feel more informed, supported, and involved in the care journey, whether you're the patient, a care partner, or both.

About Communication and Support

- Who is the main provider overseeing care?
- What are the roles of the different people on the care team?
- Who can I talk to if I have questions or feel confused about the plan?
- How often do care team rounds happen, and can I be there?
- Can someone help explain things in a way that's easier to understand?
- Are there interpreter services or language support available if we need them?
- What's the best way to get updates if I can't be at the bedside?

About Emotional Well-being

- Are there support services available for stress, fear, or emotional overwhelm?
- Can I speak with a social worker, chaplain, or mental health professional?
- How can I support my own well-being while I'm here?
- Are there quiet spaces, relaxation resources, or comfort items available?
- What can I do if I feel emotionally exhausted or unsure how to cope?
- Are there programs like art therapy, music therapy, or healing touch?

Daily Updates

Date:

Patient's Condition:
_____
_____
_____

Treatments and Procedures:
_____
_____
_____
_____

Milestones and Progress:
_____
_____
_____

Daily Goals:
_____
_____
_____

Notes:
_____
_____
_____
_____

Questions for the Medical Team

Date:

Questions Asked:
_____
_____
_____
_____
_____
_____
_____

Answers Provided:
_____
_____
_____
_____
_____
_____

Follow-Up Questions:
_____
_____
_____
_____
_____
_____

Daily Updates

Date:

Patient's Condition:
_____
_____
_____

Treatments and Procedures:
_____
_____
_____
_____

Milestones and Progress:
_____
_____
_____

Daily Goals:
_____
_____
_____

Notes:
_____
_____
_____
_____

Questions for the Medical Team

Date:

Questions Asked:
_____
_____
_____
_____
_____
_____
_____

Answers Provided:
_____
_____
_____
_____
_____
_____
_____

Follow-Up Questions:
_____
_____
_____
_____
_____
_____

Daily Wellness & Progress Tracker

Date:

Patient's Condition:
_____
_____
_____

Treatments and Procedures:
_____
_____
_____
_____

Milestones and Progress:
_____
_____
_____

Daily Goals:
_____
_____
_____

Notes:
_____
_____
_____
_____

Questions for the Medical Team

Date:

Questions Asked:
_____
_____
_____
_____
_____
_____
_____

Answers Provided:
_____
_____
_____
_____
_____
_____

Follow-Up Questions:
_____
_____
_____
_____
_____
_____

Daily Wellness & Progress Tracker

Date:

Patient's Condition:
_____
_____
_____

Treatments and Procedures:
_____
_____
_____
_____

Milestones and Progress:
_____
_____
_____

Daily Goals:
_____
_____
_____

Notes:
_____
_____
_____
_____
_____

Questions for the Medical Team

Date:

Questions Asked:
_____
_____
_____
_____
_____
_____
_____

Answers Provided:
_____
_____
_____
_____
_____
_____

Follow-Up Questions:
_____
_____
_____
_____
_____
_____
_____

Daily Wellness & Progress Tracker

Date:

Patient's Condition:
_____
_____
_____

Treatments and Procedures:
_____
_____
_____
_____

Milestones and Progress:
_____
_____
_____

Daily Goals:
_____
_____
_____

Notes:
_____
_____
_____
_____

Questions for the Medical Team

Date:

Questions Asked:
_____
_____
_____
_____
_____
_____
_____

Answers Provided:
_____
_____
_____
_____
_____
_____
_____

Follow-Up Questions:
_____
_____
_____
_____
_____
_____
_____

Daily Wellness & Progress Tracker

Date:

Patient's Condition:
_____
_____
_____

Treatments and Procedures:
_____
_____
_____
_____
_____

Milestones and Progress:
_____
_____
_____

Daily Goals:
_____
_____
_____

Notes:
_____
_____
_____
_____

Questions for the Medical Team

Date:

Questions Asked:
_____
_____
_____
_____
_____
_____
_____

Answers Provided:
_____
_____
_____
_____
_____
_____

Follow-Up Questions:
_____
_____
_____
_____
_____
_____

Daily Wellness & Progress Tracker

Date:

Patient's Condition:
___
___
___

Treatments and Procedures:
___
___
___
___

Milestones and Progress:
___
___
___

Daily Goals:
___
___
___

Notes:
___
___
___
___

Questions for the Medical Team

Date:

Questions Asked:
_____
_____
_____
_____
_____
_____
_____

Answers Provided:
_____
_____
_____
_____
_____
_____
_____

Follow-Up Questions:
_____
_____
_____
_____
_____
_____
_____

Daily Wellness & Progress Tracker

Date:

Patient's Condition:
_____
_____
_____

Treatments and Procedures:
_____
_____
_____
_____

Milestones and Progress:
_____
_____
_____

Daily Goals:
_____
_____
_____

Notes:
_____
_____
_____
_____

Questions for the Medical Team

Date:

Questions Asked:
_____
_____
_____
_____
_____
_____
_____

Answers Provided:
_____
_____
_____
_____
_____
_____

Follow-Up Questions:
_____
_____
_____
_____
_____
_____

Daily Wellness & Progress Tracker

Date:

Patient's Condition:
___
___
___

Treatments and Procedures:
___
___
___
___

Milestones and Progress:
___
___
___

Daily Goals:
___
___
___

Notes:
___
___
___
___

Questions for the Medical Team

Date:

Questions Asked:
_____
_____
_____
_____
_____
_____

Answers Provided:
_____
_____
_____
_____
_____
_____

Follow-Up Questions:
_____
_____
_____
_____
_____
_____

Daily Wellness & Progress Tracker

Date:

Patient's Condition:
_____
_____
_____

Treatments and Procedures:
_____
_____
_____
_____

Milestones and Progress:
_____
_____
_____

Daily Goals:
_____
_____
_____

Notes:
_____
_____
_____
_____

Questions for the Medical Team

Date:

Questions Asked:
_____
_____
_____
_____
_____
_____
_____

Answers Provided:
_____
_____
_____
_____
_____
_____
_____

Follow-Up Questions:
_____
_____
_____
_____
_____
_____
_____

Daily Wellness & Progress Tracker

Date:

Patient's Condition:
___
___
___

Treatments and Procedures:
___
___
___
___

Milestones and Progress:
___
___
___

Daily Goals:
___
___
___

Notes:
___
___
___
___

Questions for the Medical Team

Date:

Questions Asked:
_____
_____
_____
_____
_____
_____
_____

Answers Provided:
_____
_____
_____
_____
_____
_____
_____

Follow-Up Questions:
_____
_____
_____
_____
_____
_____
_____

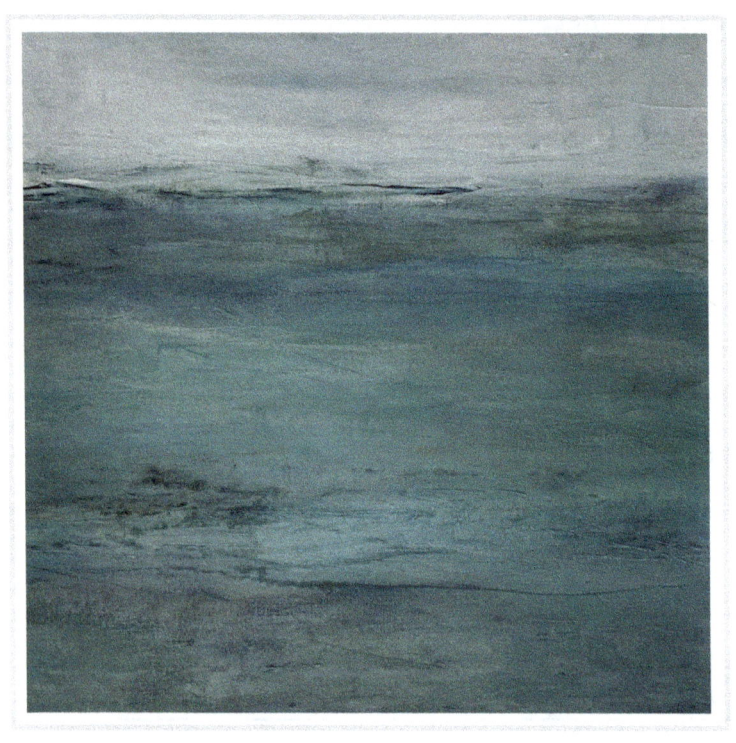

*This moment is part of the story,
but it is not the whole story.*

-Unknown

Caring for Yourself During a Hospital Stay

Being in the hospital, whether as a patient or a loved one, can feel overwhelming. It's important to recognize that you're doing your best and to take small steps to care for yourself along the way.

Taking Small Breaks

Give yourself a few moments to recharge throughout the day. You don't have to leave your space. Try stretching, deep breathing, or using a mindfulness app. Some hospitals may offer relaxation programs, music therapy, or other support services, so ask your care team what's available.

Focus on What You Can Control

When things feel uncertain, small actions can help create a sense of stability:

- Take deep breaths to calm your body and mind.
- Write down questions or thoughts to stay organized.
- Engage in a quiet activity, like listening to music, reading, or journaling.

Stay Connected with Support

If friends or family can help, let them. Accepting support, even in small ways, can relieve pressure. Many people find it helpful to set up group updates or use a website like **CaringBridge.com** to keep loved ones informed.

Acknowledge Your Efforts

You are doing your best in a difficult situation. Sometimes, a simple reminder that you're showing up and doing what you can is enough to restore confidence and strength. Even small steps can provide clarity and comfort during this time.

Mindfulness and Relaxation Exercises

Deep Breathing Exercise

Place one hand on your chest and the other on your belly. Take a deep breath in through your nose, feeling your belly expand, then slowly exhale through your mouth. Try this for a few minutes to calm your nervous system and regain focus.

Grounding Technique

When you feel overwhelmed, focus on your surroundings to ground yourself. Identify five things you can see, four things you can touch, three things you can hear, two things you can smell, and one thing you can taste. This technique can help shift your attention away from stress and back to the present moment.

Progressive Muscle Relaxation

Starting with your toes, tense each muscle group in your body for a few seconds, then release. Gradually move up through your legs, abdomen, arms, and face, releasing tension as you go. This technique helps relieve physical stress and can make you feel more relaxed.

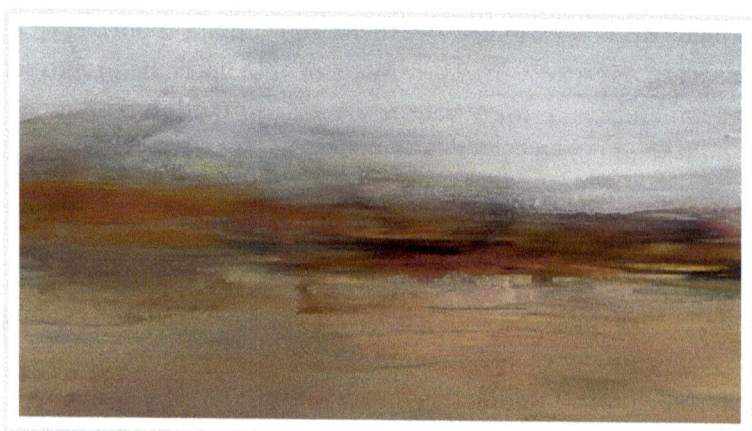

Emotional Reflections

Caring for yourself emotionally is just as important as physical recovery. Use this space however feels best for you. Whether that's writing, drawing, or simply taking a moment to pause.

Consider These Prompts to Guide Your Reflection

- How am I feeling today? (physically, emotionally, mentally?)
- What's one small thing that brought me comfort?
- What's something I want to let go of today?
- What's within my control right now?
- What's something I'm grateful for?
- A message of encouragement to myself or a loved one.

Use the following pages however you like. Write, reflect, or express in whatever way feels right for you.

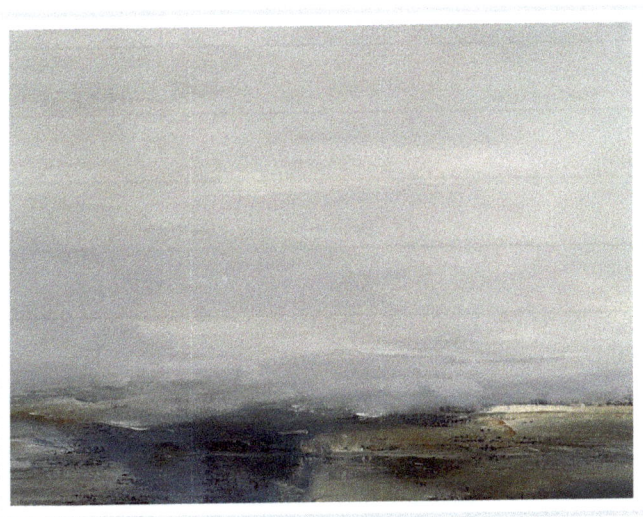

Date: _____

Progress is not linear. Every step matters.

Date: _____

*Healing isn't just physical- it's emotional too.
Be gentle with yourself.*

Date: _____

_____
_____
_____
_____
_____
_____
_____
_____
_____
_____
_____
_____
_____
_____
_____
_____

You are worthy of kindness, including from yourself.

Date: _____

_____
_____
_____
_____
_____
_____
_____
_____
_____
_____
_____
_____
_____
_____
_____
_____
_____

A little hope each day adds up to healing.

Date: _____

_____
_____
_____
_____
_____
_____
_____
_____
_____
_____
_____
_____
_____
_____
_____
_____
_____

Hold onto hope. Even the smallest light can guide you through the darkest moments.

Date:_____

_____
_____
_____
_____
_____
_____
_____
_____
_____
_____
_____
_____
_____
_____
_____

Take a deep breath. You are here, and that is enough.

Date: _____

_____

_____

_____

_____

_____

_____

_____

_____

_____

_____

_____

_____

_____

_____

_____

You are not alone. There are people who care about you.

Date: _____

It's okay to rest. Healing takes time.

Date: _____

Small steps forward still count as progress.

Date: _____

Your thoughts and emotions are valid.

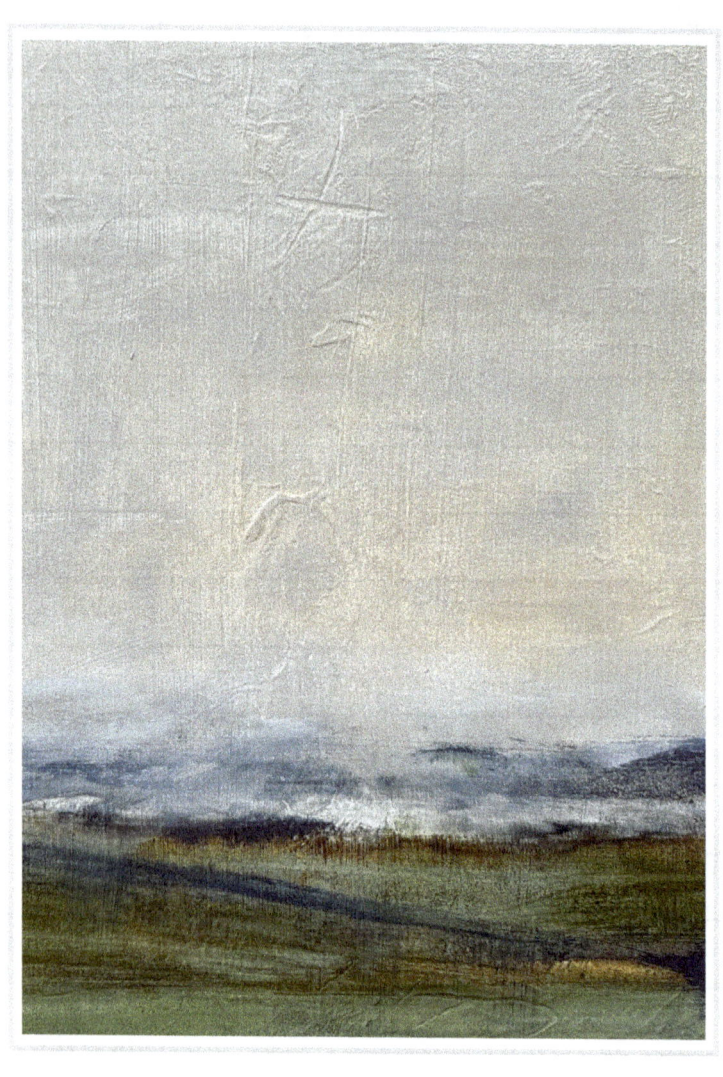

The hard days are what make you stronger.

- Aly Raisman

Date: _____

_____
_____
_____
_____
_____
_____
_____
_____
_____
_____
_____
_____
_____
_____
_____
_____

It's okay to rest. Healing takes time.

Date:_____

_____
_____
_____
_____
_____
_____
_____
_____
_____
_____
_____
_____
_____
_____
_____

Give yourself the same kindness you would give to a friend.

Date: _____

_____
_____
_____
_____
_____
_____
_____
_____
_____
_____
_____
_____
_____
_____
_____
_____
_____
_____

When you can't see the whole path, just take the next small step.

Date: _____

Let go of what you can't control, and focus on what you can.

Take life one breath at a time; you're doing better than you think.

- Unknown

Messages and Notes for Your Loved One

Please use this space for supportive notes or updates that can be shared with your loved one during or after recovery. Consider writing each entry as if you're speaking directly to them. You might start by explaining what brought them to the hospital or the ICU, then share updates on their condition, treatments, and any progress they're making. Including personal messages or news from outside the hospital can help them feel connected to the world beyond their hospital bed, easing any sense of lost time.

Date:

_____
_____
_____
_____
_____
_____

Date:

_____
_____
_____
_____
_____
_____

Messages and Notes for Your Loved One

Date:

_____
_____
_____
_____
_____
_____

Date:

_____
_____
_____
_____
_____
_____

Date:

_____
_____
_____
_____
_____
_____

Messages and Notes for Your Loved One

Date:

_____
_____
_____
_____
_____
_____

Date:

_____
_____
_____
_____
_____
_____

Date:

_____
_____
_____
_____
_____
_____

Messages and Notes for Your Loved One

Date:

_____
_____
_____
_____
_____
_____
_____

Date:

_____
_____
_____
_____
_____
_____
_____

Date:

_____
_____
_____
_____
_____
_____
_____

Messages and Notes for Your Loved One

Date:

_____
_____
_____
_____
_____
_____
_____

Date:

_____
_____
_____
_____
_____
_____
_____

Date:

_____
_____
_____
_____
_____
_____
_____

Messages and Notes for Your Loved One

Date:
_____
_____
_____
_____
_____
_____

Date:
_____
_____
_____
_____
_____
_____

Date:
_____
_____
_____
_____
_____
_____

Messages and Notes for Your Loved One

Date:

_____
_____
_____
_____
_____
_____
_____

Date:

_____
_____
_____
_____
_____
_____
_____

Date:

_____
_____
_____
_____
_____
_____
_____

Messages and Notes for Your Loved One

Date:
_____
_____
_____
_____
_____
_____

Date:
_____
_____
_____
_____
_____
_____

Date:
_____
_____
_____
_____
_____
_____

Messages and Notes for Your Loved One

Date:

_____
_____
_____
_____
_____
_____
_____

Date:

_____
_____
_____
_____
_____
_____
_____

Date:

_____
_____
_____
_____
_____
_____
_____

Messages and Notes for Your Loved One

Date:

_____
_____
_____
_____
_____
_____

Date:

_____
_____
_____
_____
_____
_____

Date:

_____
_____
_____
_____
_____
_____

Messages and Notes for Your Loved One

Date:
_____
_____
_____
_____
_____
_____

Date:
_____
_____
_____
_____
_____
_____

Date:
_____
_____
_____
_____
_____
_____

Messages and Notes for Your Loved One

Date:
_____
_____
_____
_____
_____
_____
_____
_____

Date:
_____
_____
_____
_____
_____
_____
_____

Date:
_____
_____
_____
_____
_____
_____
_____

Messages and Notes for Your Loved One

Date:

_____
_____
_____
_____
_____
_____

Date:

_____
_____
_____
_____
_____
_____

Date:

_____
_____
_____
_____
_____
_____

Messages and Notes for Your Loved One

Date:

_____
_____
_____
_____
_____
_____

Date:

_____
_____
_____
_____
_____
_____

Date:

_____
_____
_____
_____
_____
_____

Patient Reflections

This section is a space for the patient to share their thoughts, wishes, or feelings if they're able to. They can write or express anything important to them, whether it's something they want to remember, hopes they have, things they're looking forward to, or simply how they're feeling in the moment.

There's no right or wrong way to use this section.
Write as much or as little as you'd like.

Date:

_____

_____

_____

_____

_____

_____

_____

_____

_____

Patient Reflections

Optional Prompt: What are you thinking about today?

Date:

_____

_____

_____

_____

_____

_____

_____

_____

_____

_____

_____

Patient Reflections

Optional Prompt: Is there anything you're looking forward to or hoping for?

Date:

Patient Reflections

Optional Prompt: What would you like your family or caregivers to know about how you're feeling?

Date:

_____

_____

_____

_____

_____

_____

_____

_____

_____

_____

_____

Patient Reflections

Optional Prompt: What has been helping you feel supported during this time?

Date:

_____

_____

_____

_____

_____

_____

_____

_____

_____

_____

Patient Reflections

Optional Prompt: Describe what you're looking forward to, no matter how small.

Date:

_____

_____

_____

_____

_____

_____

_____

_____

_____

_____

_____

Patient Reflections

Optional Prompt: Write about a favorite memory that helps you feel strong.

Date:

_____

_____

_____

_____

_____

_____

_____

_____

_____

_____

_____

Patient Reflections

Optional Prompt: Write about something or someone that brings you comfort right now.

Date:

_____

_____

_____

_____

_____

_____

_____

_____

_____

_____

_____

_____

Hospital Support Services Available During Your Stay

Hospitals offer a range of support services to help patients and families navigate care, address practical concerns, and find emotional and spiritual support.

Spiritual Care Chaplains provide emotional and spiritual support to patients and families, regardless of faith or belief. They are available for beside visits, private conversations, or simply as a source of comfort during uncertain times.

Social Workers Social workers assist with practical needs, including discharge planning, accessing financial or community resources, and addressing concerns related to care and recovery.

Case Managers Case managers help coordinate care, manage transitions between hospital and home or rehabilitation, and ensure that complex medical and logistical needs are met.

Palliative Care Palliative care teams focus on relieving symptoms, pain, and stress in patients with serious illnesses. They provide emotional and spiritual support, help families understand treatment options, and ensure that care aligns with patient goals. Palliative care is available at any stage of an illness and can be provided alongside active treatments.

These services exist to support you. Don't hesitate to ask your care team how to connect with them.

Community & Online Support

Caring Bridge A free online tool for families to communicate updates with friends and loved ones, reducing the burden of repeated messages. www.caringbridge.org

Lotsa Helping Hands A platform to coordinate care and organize support for patients and families. www.lotsahelpinghands.com

Meal Train A tool for organizing meal deliveries and support for patient and families. www.mealtrain.com

HealthWell Foundation Recognized as one of America's most efficient charities, they provide grants to reduce barriers to care for under insured Americans. www.Healthwellfoundation.org

The ARCH National Respite Network A service to help caregivers and professionals locate respite services in their community. www.archrespite.org

National Respite Coalition A service that advocates for preserving and promoting respite policy and programs at the national, state, and local levels. www.nhchc.org

AARP Programs and Services Provides support for food, housing, health and employment in your area. AARP's Caregiver Resource Center offers a variety of resources for caregivers and families. www.aarp.org

American Cancer Society Programs and Services Offers free lodging, transportation to treatment, breast cancer support, online communities, and free family and patient programs. www.cancer.org

Take life one breath at a time; you're doing better than you think.

- Unknown

After the ICU: Continuing Recovery with This Diary

As your loved one begins to heal beyond the ICU, this journal can offer a meaningful space to reflect on the progress made and the challenges you've faced together.

Transitioning to a step down or general medical floor often brings a mix of relief and uncertainty. While the level of care may feel different, this step forward signals greater stability and readiness for the next phase of recovery.

Ways to Use the Journal in Recovery

Celebrate Milestones

- Revisit earlier entries to recognize how far your loved one has come. It can help you stay grounded in the progress already made.

Reflect Together

- Reading entries aloud can help fill in memory gaps and support emotional healing, especially if your loved one doesn't recall parts of their ICU stay.

Seek Support

- If symptoms related to Post-Intensive Care Syndrome (PICS) persist, resources like social workers, nurse coaches, and PICS clinics can help. Visit POSTICU.org or ICUdelerium.org for more information and support.

If you feel overwhelmed, don't hesitate to reach out. Your care team understands this transition and is here to support you every step of the way.

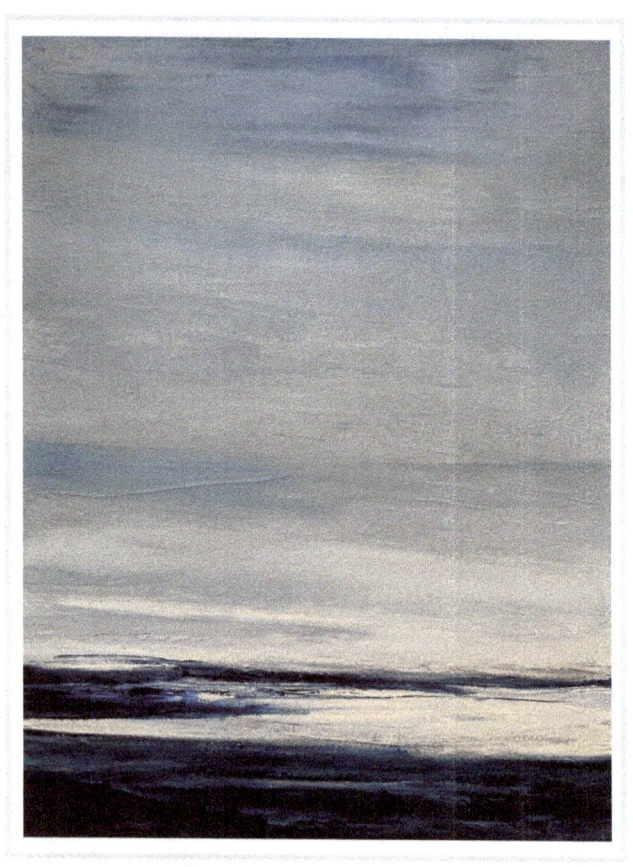

Healing takes time, but every step forward is progress.

- Unknown

A Note of Gratitude

Take a moment to recognize someone who made a difference in your care: a nurse, doctor, therapist, or anyone who helped you feel supported. Tear it out and give it to them as a simple way to share your gratitude and acknowledge their care.

Name (if known): _____

Role or Unit: _____

What they did that stood out: _____

_____

_____

A Note of Gratitude

Take a moment to recognize someone who made a difference in your care: a nurse, doctor, therapist, or anyone who helped you feel supported. Tear it out and give it to them as a simple way to share your gratitude and acknowledge their care.

Name (if known): _____

Role or Unit: _____

What they did that stood out: _____

_____

_____

"Getting to Know Me"

Please call me: _____

My family members are: _____
_____
_____

They can be reached at: _____
_____

My hobbies are: _____
_____
_____
_____

I'm looking forward to getting home for: _____
_____
_____

My favorite TV shows, sports teams, or music are: _____
_____
_____

Things that make me smile: _____
_____
_____

More about me: _____
_____
_____
_____

Thank you for caring for me!

Notes

Notes

Notes

Notes

Notes

Notes

Notes

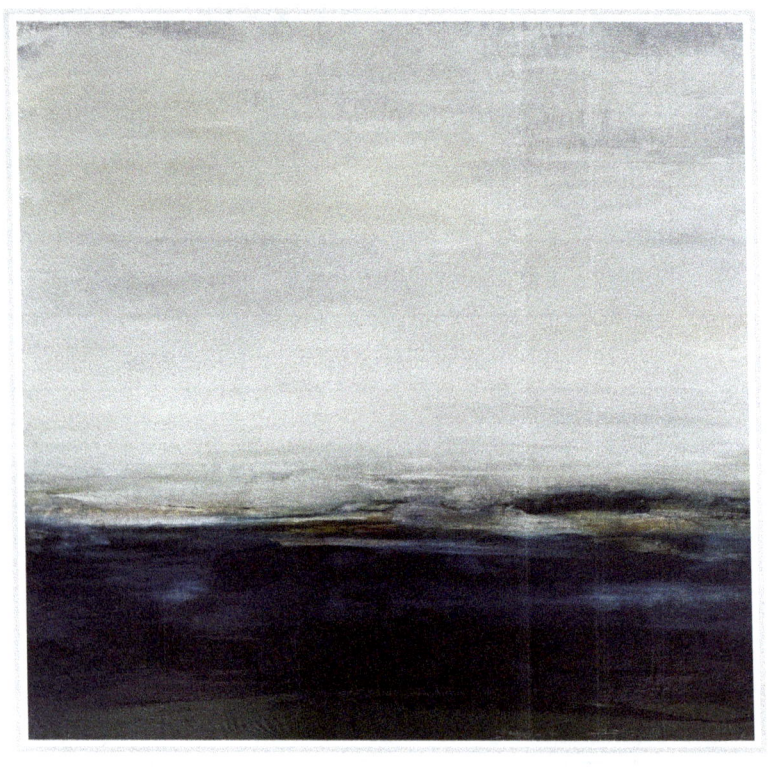

*Courage doesn't always roar. Sometimes courage is
the quiet voice at the end of the day saying,
'I will try again tomorrow.'*

- Mary Ann Radmacher

Notes

Notes

Notes

Notes

About the Author

Nicole Cromwell is a nurse with twenty-five years of critical care experience, including many years supporting patients and families in intensive care settings. Her time in the ICU shaped her deep understanding of the emotional and practical challenges that come with a loved one's critical illness.

Now based in Carmel, California, Nicole has shifted from bedside nursing to a full-time art practice. Her clinical background and creative work come together in this journal, offering families a gentle, supportive resource during a challenging time.

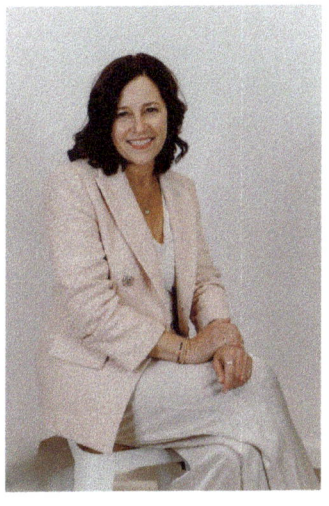

Thank you for spending time with this journal. Whether you are a patient, a care partner, or a member of the hospital staff, your experience matters deeply to me. This journal was created to support healing during some of life's most difficult moments, and I'm always looking for ways to make it more helpful and compassionate.

Please take a moment to share your feedback by scanning the QR code below. The survey is completely anonymous, open to anyone who used or interacted with the journal, and takes less than 2 minutes to complete.

www.icudiary.com
www.hospitalwellnessjournal.com
www.nicolecromwellart.com

www.ingramcontent.com/pod-product-compliance
Lightning Source LLC
Chambersburg PA
CBHW070642030426
42337CB00020B/4129